Eliminate Your Varicose and Spider Veins Now!

Dr. Peter Ursel

Copyright ©2013 by Peter Ursel M.D.

All rights reserved. No portion of this book may be reproduced--mechanically, electronically, or by any other means without the expressed written permission of the author.

Published by Peter Ursel M.D. Lindsay, Ontario

All rights reserved

ISBN-13: 978-1490547152

ISBN-10: 1490547150

The Publisher has strived to be as accurate and complete as possible in the creation of this book.

This book is not intended for use as a source of medical or legal advice. All readers are advised to seek services of competent professionals in the medical field.

In practical advice books, like anything else in life, there are no guarantees of medical cures. Readers are cautioned to rely on their own judgment about their individual circumstances to act accordingly.

While all attempts have been made to verify information provided in this publication, the Publisher assumes no responsibility for errors, omissions, or contrary interpretation of the subject matter herein. Any perceived slights of specific persons, peoples, or organizations are unintentional.

For more information, please visit www.doctorursel.com, www.veinbook.com or www.whitbyveinclinic.com

Table of Contents

Chapter 1	Introduction	7
Chapter 2	What Causes Varicose Veins?	11
Chapter 3	What Are The Different Types Of Leg Veins?	19
Chapter 4	How Can I Treat My Veins At Home?	25
Chapter 5	What Types Of Vein Treatments Are Available?	35
Chapter 6	What Can Happen Without Treatment?	45
Chapter 7	What Are The Possible Complications Of Treatment?	51
Chapter 8	How Are Leg Veins Evaluated?	59
Chapter 9	Other Common Questions	65
Chapter 10	Common Myths About Leg Veins	75
Chapter 11	Case Studies Of Successful Treatments	87
Chapter 12	Summary	99
About Dr Ursel		101

Chapter 1
Introduction

In this concise book, my goal is to give you the information you need to eliminate unsightly leg veins in the safest and quickest manner possible.

I have been treating leg veins for more than 20 years, and I have seen firsthand how leg veins can cause a considerable amount of pain and cosmetic distress. The scope of this problem is huge, as abnormal leg veins affect 1 out of every 4 adults, most of these being women.

However, there is good news! During my last 20 years treating leg veins, there's been an explosion of amazing new technologies. These technologies have made the diagnosis and treatment of veins incredibly safe and effective. Today there is no need to suffer with leg veins or to undergo risky and dangerous treatments.

In this book, you are going to learn the essential facts you need to know if you suffer with varicose veins and want to get them safely and effectively treated.

First, you will learn about the underlying cause of varicose veins and then you will discover the 4 basic types of treatments that are currently available on the market.

I will show you what can happen if you leave your veins alone and do nothing, and explain the possible complications of treatment.

I will walk you through the assessment process involved and discuss what you should look for in a vein clinic. I will go over several case studies of people that have had their veins treated and discuss the outcomes they had. I will answer the most common questions I get about veins and will discuss common myths about leg veins. You will finally learn the truth about many of these common misconceptions.

My goal is to help you make an informed choice to eliminate your unsightly and possibly dangerous leg veins. With accurate assessment and up to date modern treatment technologies, it's never been easier or safer to eliminate your troublesome leg veins!

Eliminate Your Varicose and Spider Veins Now!

Dr. Peter Ursel

Chapter 2
What Causes Varicose Veins?

Varicose veins are very common, affecting up to 25% of women and 15% of men. In this section, you'll learn about the underlying cause of most leg veins and also about the aggravating factors that make veins worse.

To understand what causes varicose veins, one must remember that there are two types of blood vessels: arteries and veins.

Arteries

Arteries bring blood down to the legs under pulsating, high pressure. The blood is under high pressure as it has just been pumped from the heart and for the most part is flowing down hill, with gravity to the lower parts of the body.

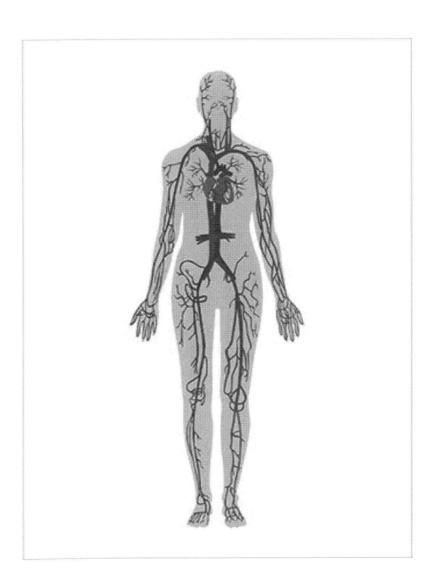

Veins, on the other hand, bring the blood to the heart from the extremities of the body, and in the legs it flows more slowly because it is flowing upwards against gravity.

To counteract the slow flow and the effect of gravity, there are special valves found inside veins. These valves keep blood flowing upwards and are found in almost all types of veins throughout the body.

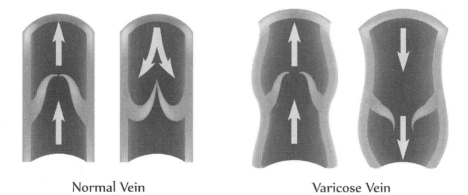

Normal Vein   Varicose Vein

The leg veins are under higher pressure so there are more valves in the leg veins. When these valves become damaged, varicose veins can form.

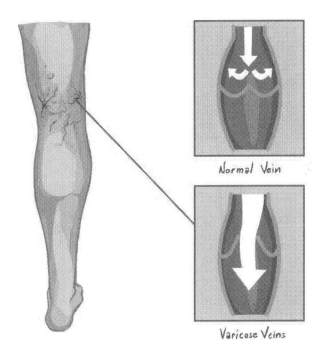

What Causes Vein Valves To Fail?

There are several causes of valve failure. The most prominent factors are probably genetics and family history.

Some people are, unfortunately, born with a hereditary weakness of valves in their veins. You can do nothing about heredity factors; however, there are other factors which aggravate varicose veins that you do have an opportunity to control.

Examples of these aggravating factors include: repetitive and heavy straining and standing for long periods of time. One of the most common causes of poor valve function is pregnancy. This aggravation comes from the increased pressure inside the veins that accompanies pregnancy. In pregnancy, there is also an increase in blood volume which further strains the valves.

The common denominator in all of these factors is that they all increase pressure inside the veins, which strains the valves, eventually leading them to failure.

Summary

Varicose veins are caused by a simple mechanical problem with the valves found inside the veins. This failure is probably caused by congenital weakness of these valves and made worse by the increased pressure found in pregnancy, heavy straining and prolonged standing.

Eliminate Your Varicose and Spider Veins Now!

Dr. Peter Ursel

Chapter 3
What Are the Different Types of Leg Veins?

There are 3 main types of visible leg veins which are all interconnected.

Varicose Veins

First there are the largest veins, the worm-like varicose veins. These can be found on all parts of the legs and in the genital area. Varicose veins can cause the greatest problems. They're known to cause skin discoloration, swelling, rashes and ulceration. The appearance of varicose veins is usually a sign of a deeper problem within the circulatory system.

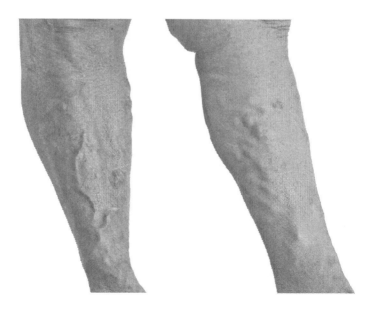

The root of the problem is usually found deep inside or high up the leg, or sometimes inside the pelvis. These veins tend to get longer with time. This lengthening often causes the veins to resemble thickened, stacked worms just under the skin.

If your varicose veins are painful it is because nerves inside the vein walls are sensitive to stretching, which occurs when the blood pools inside of them.

Green Veins or Reticular Veins

Second, are the reticular or green veins.

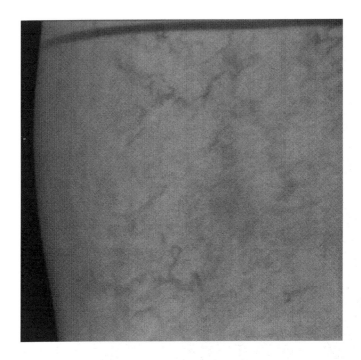

Smaller than varicose veins, reticular or green veins are more visible in people with light colored or thin skin. These veins do not usually bulge, but they can be unsightly for those with very thin skin. Reticular or green veins are branches of the larger veins that feed them. They become enlarged if they are attached to varicose veins, and when enlarged this is evidence of a deeper problem within the system.

Reticular veins warrant attention because they are not only unsightly, but they lead to surface capillaries. If the pressure inside reticular veins is high, it will cause surface capillaries to enlarge, turning them into spider veins.

Spider Veins

Spider veins are the most common veins. They cause considerable cosmetic distress and, in some people, they can be quite uncomfortable.

They can range in color from bright red to dark blue. Spider veins branch off of reticular veins. They become worse with time and the increased pressure inside of reticular veins. While spider veins are mainly a cosmetic concern, in some people, they can be painful with occasional bleeding, if they are connected to high-pressure deep vessels and become traumatized.

Dr. Peter Ursel

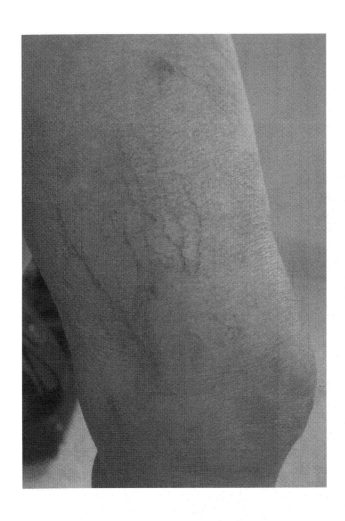

It's important to realize that spider veins are fed by deeper green or reticular veins. This information is a key to the successful elimination of spider veins. They are almost always eliminated by, first, closing down their feeding reticular veins.

Summary

There are three basic types of veins:

1. The large varicose veins.

2. The middle sized green or reticular veins.

3. The smallest spider veins.

All of these types of veins are important and need to be treated in a customized fashion.

Dr. Peter Ursel

Chapter 4
How Can I Treat My Veins At Home?

At home, there are several things you can do to improve symptoms and the visible appearance of your leg veins. When applying these particular home treatments, you will also prevent your leg veins from getting worse.

Exercise

The most important measure you can take is getting regular exercise. Truthfully, all types of exercise will help. However, there are some exercises that are better than others, and there are some exercises that should be avoided.

The best exercise for leg veins is walking. Walking is good because the activity in the calf muscles pushes the blood up your legs. This massaging action also helps to relieve swelling in the lower legs. For the same reason, cycling is an excellent form of exercise as well if you have leg veins.

Dr. Peter Ursel

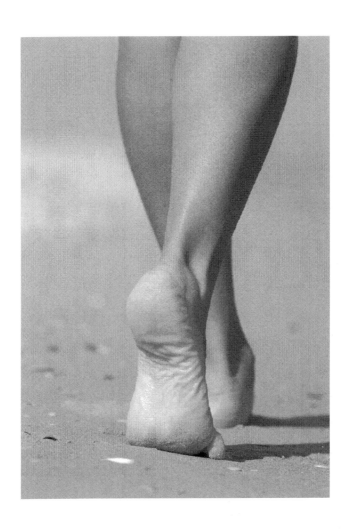

Swimming is another excellent exercise because your body is horizontal when you are swimming. This helps drain blood more easily from your legs and return it to the heart. It is also a very smooth action. Some exercises, especially the pounding types, push blood down the legs, making it more difficult to get adequate leg vein drainage. Therefore, walking, cycling and swimming are ideal activities to aid in treating varicose veins.

As an added bonus, exercise also helps your bowel function. This is important because, if you're constipated there is usually a lot of straining involved. Straining due to constipation causes increased pressure in the pelvic veins, which increases congestion in varicose veins. So, having good bowel function is important and it is enhanced by regular exercise.

Please note: there are certain types of exercise that should be avoided. Heavy weight lifting causes straining and this straining pushes down on pelvic veins. This increases pressure in leg veins, causing more swelling of veins in the legs.

Weight Loss

If you suffer with any type of varicose veins, you should also attempt losing weight. Weight loss causes less pressure to be placed on pelvic veins. If there is a lot of abdominal fat, this impedes drainage of blood from pelvis. When blood is not draining properly from the pelvis, it causes congestion in leg veins. So, when you lose weight you get decreased pressure in the pelvis.

When you lose weight there is less fat around the varicose veins, especially the thigh veins. This should be noted if you're considering any type of varicose vein treatments, because it is much easier for the doctor to access and treat the veins.

It also makes it less likely that you will experience complications after your treatments. Losing weight will also make it much easier to apply compression bandages and stockings because the legs are slimmer. There is also less of a chance of infection after treatment if there is a smaller amount of fat tissue in the vein area. Weight loss should be considered, if it is an issue, for all varicose vein patients.

Compression Stockings

Compression stockings, or support hose are suggested if you have varicose veins. If you have severe varicose veins and chronic venous insufficiency, high compression stockings in the range of 40-50 mm of mercury are required.

However, lower compression stockings in the range of 10-20 mm of mercury can work quite nicely; especially, if your vein disease is not too severe. The advantage of these lower compression stockings is that they are easier to put on, making it more likely that you'll use them on a regular basis.

The question always arises, whether you should have full leg stockings or knee high stockings? Full leg stockings are probably better; however, they are more difficult to put on, making it less likely that you'll wear them regularly.

If you are hesitant about wearing stockings using knee high stockings is preferable to no stockings at all. Compression stockings can be used to dramatically improve the symptoms that occur from varicose veins. They can prevent worsening of leg veins, especially if treatment is not possible due to medical or financial reasons.

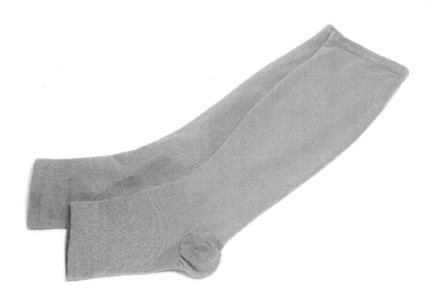

Leg Elevation

Leg elevation can help to improve varicose vein symptoms.

The legs can be elevated after prolonged exercise and can also be elevated when you're resting.

For example, if you're watching television, it is good to elevate your legs on a pillow and then do exercises to improve circulation in your lower legs. These exercises can include extending your ankles and bending your knees back and forth. These measures can help to relieve congestion and discomfort in your legs.

Nutritional Measures

Having a high fiber diet is important because it helps with bowel functions. As mentioned earlier, good bowel function decreases the amount of pressure placed on pelvic veins.

You may also want to consider adding some extra nutritional supplements to your diet. Antioxidant vitamins such as vitamins A, C, E and selenium are good for blood vessel health. In general, they can help support the health of the vein walls. Stronger vein walls help to minimize the distention of the veins, therefore improving vein health.

An herbal treatment, known as horse chestnut, has also been used for centuries. This has been shown to help many people that have varicose veins. Consider horse chestnut treatment as an option in your nutritional approach to treating veins.

Things to Avoid

There are certain things you should avoid if you have varicose veins, and these things are fairly obvious. Inactivity is the opposite of exercise, and it can definitely make leg veins worse. In addition, if you work standing in the same position for long periods of time, this may cause worsening pain and congestion of varicose veins.

Many people who have standing jobs tend to have more problems with varicose veins. They should, at least, consider using support hose. Also, try to avoid prolonged standing, if possible. If you do have this type of job, make sure that you walk around. Moving your feet and ankles periodically will help to improve the blood flow in the legs.

Summary

There are several measures you can take to aid in the treatment of leg veins. You can exercise, lose weight, use compression stockings, elevate your legs whenever possible, take supportive nutritional supplements, and avoid certain factors. If you take some or all of these measures, you'll be less likely to have complications from your varicose veins, and you'll have less discomfort in your legs. If you do have any vein treatments or procedures, you are going to be better prepared and less likely to have complications from these procedures. All of these measures help to improve your general health, so they are highly recommended.

Eliminate Your Varicose and Spider Veins Now!

Dr. Peter Ursel

Chapter 5
What Types Of Vein Treatments Are Available?

In this section we will discuss the various types of vein treatments that are currently available. Additionally, in order to give you a better understanding of the various treatments available, I will explain in which circumstances they are used.

Four Types of Treatments

There are four types of treatments that clinics and doctors provide for leg veins. There are:

1. Surgical treatments.

2. Injection sclerotherapy treatments.

3. Endovenous procedures (going inside the veins using special catheters).

4. Surface lasers (used from the outside of the body to work on blood vessels).

So, let's go over each of them in detail.

Surgical Treatments

There are two types of surgical options available. There is traditional stripping and ligation, and a procedure called ambulatory phlebectomy.

As mentioned stripping and ligation is the traditional treatment. It is usually done in a hospital setting under general anesthesia. There is usually an incision made in the groin and other incisions are made on the inner aspect of the leg. These incisions are made to remove the greater saphenous vein.

The incision in the groin allows for ligation at the top of the vein and removal of the vein. The incision in the leg allows for the placement of a probe inside the vein. Following this, the vein is pulled or stripped out. Hence, the treatment name.

The second type of surgical treatment is called ambulatory phlebectomy. This treatment is mostly done on smaller surface blood vessels that are usually bulging. It is done under local anesthetic by administering the anesthetic in the areas around the vein. The veins are removed with special hooks. Then afterwards, pressure is put on the vein area.

The incisions are extremely small, and they are usually created with special needles. Usually there is minimal scarring because the incisions are so small and there is minimal trauma.

However, there is the possibility of some bleeding after treatment.

Injection Sclerotherapy

The second class of treatment is injection sclerotherapy. There are two types of injection sclerotherapy. First, there is traditional injection sclerotherapy, which is done with liquid solutions. Second, there is a newer treatment called foam sclerotherapy.

Liquid sclerotherapy is done by injecting special solutions right into the veins. A traditional example of liquid sclerotherapy would be a saline injection. Liquid sclerotherapy treatments are used on smaller types of blood vessels. There are also other types of solutions that can be used which are stronger. These solutions include iodine, polydocanol, and sodium tetra-decyl sulphate.

The second type of treatment is a newer treatment than liquid sclerotherapy called foam sclerotherapy. A foam solution is created by mixing the sclerosing solution with either CO_2 or room air in a special type of syringe.

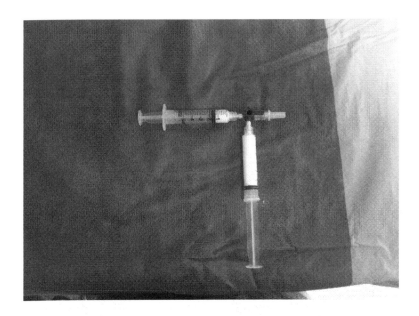

The result is that a white-colored foam forms. The foam is then injected into the targeted veins. Interestingly, the entire process can be seen on an ultrasound. The solution can be followed into the deeper blood vessels. The advantage of the foam sclerotherapy treatment is that the foam stays in contact with vein walls longer, which allows for an enhanced effect.

Also, the foam acts as a stronger solution than if it was used in just liquid form. The foam can be used on many different types of veins; from smaller spider vessels to large saphenous veins. Foam sclerotherapy is an excellent treatment and is now being used more frequently because it is very safe and has minimal side effects.

Endovenous Procedures

Endovenous procedures are the third type of treatment we will discuss. Endovenous procedures are treatments in which a special catheter is placed inside the targeted vein. The treatment device is then placed inside this catheter for the particular type of treatment being performed.

There are three main types of endovenous procedures. One type is endovenous laser treatment (EVLT). This treatment involves a laser fiber being placed inside of a catheter, which is inside of the big vein.

Then, the area around the vein is frozen with a special local anesthetic.

Next, the leg is elevated and all blood is squeezed out of the vein. The laser is turned on and pulled out of the vein, allowing the closure of the vein from the beginning to the end of the vein. The vein is then sealed or closed by the heat from the laser inside the vein. This is the traditional type of endovenous laser treatment.

Another treatment is radio frequency closure (RF closure). This treatment is similar to EVLT, however, a special probe is used that uses radio frequency as an energy source, rather than using a laser. Radio frequency closure gives results similar to EVLT and is very effective.

The third type of endovenous treatment is the Clarivein system. This endovenous treatment is very new and uses a special catheter just like EVLT. However, instead of using a laser, a special wire is placed inside the catheter that spins rapidly. At the same time as the rapid spinning, it scratches the inside of the vein and a solution is injected through the end of the catheter.

The advantage of this treatment is that it does not require a local anesthetic, there is a quick recovery time, and there is less discomfort afterward. The results are very similar to EVLT and the RF closure. The disadvantages to the Clarivein system are that it is fairly new, and long-term studies have not been done. Also, some people can react to the solution, a problem that cannot occur with the other 2 types of endovenous treatments.

Laser Treatments of Surface Veins

The fourth type of treatment uses surface lasers. These surface lasers are roughly divided into two different categories. One category is intense pulse light or broadband light. The second category is diode lasers.

Intense pulse light or broadband light is used on very tiny blood vessels where there is a mesh of vessels visible. This treatment is used very commonly on facial blood vessels and smaller leg vessels, or vessels found on other parts of body. It is a very good treatment however is limited to use on very tiny blood vessels.

Diode lasers, on the other hand, can be used on slightly larger blood vessels. These are lasers that go right over the vein and use a different type of laser light to carry out the treatment. The disadvantage of using a diode laser is that it can discolor or lighten the skin. It must be used carefully on patients with darker pigmentations.

Combination Therapy

It's important to remember that these treatments can be used in different combinations. Often surgeries and injections are used together. Endovenous procedures and injections can be used together or any other combination of the above. Sometimes sclerotherapy is used on bigger blood vessels and tiny blood vessels are cleaned up with laser or BBL treatments.

The Best Treatments

So, what treatment is best? The answer to this question depends a lot on the doctor's preferences and training. Many doctors are trained to do one type of treatment. Surgeons tend to favor surgical treatments, and often, they do not offer sclerotherapy as part of the package. (The type of treatment depends a lot on the type of vein). The best doctors and the best centers are going to have many different treatment options at their disposal. They will customize them as per the type of veins and the particular problem(s).

Summary

There are four basic types of vein treatments:

1. Surgical
2. Injection sclerotherapy
3. Endovenous treatments
4. Surface lasers

These treatments can be used in several different combinations depending on the type of veins and the center at which you are having your veins treated.

It is to be hoped that this section has given you a good survey of the different types of treatments available.

Dr. Peter Ursel

Chapter 6
What Can Happen Without Treatment?

If you leave your veins alone and don't get treatment, several things can occur. In a small number of people the veins will not get any worse and nothing serious will happen. It is difficult to tell which people this will occur in. What happens in many cases over time is that the veins just simply get gradually worse in appearance.

In many people the veins initially are not uncomfortable however, over time they become increasingly painful and unsightly.

Phlebitis

If veins are left untreated there is a higher risk of phlebitis, which is a painful inflammation of the veins. Superficial phlebitis or inflammation of the surface veins can lead to the progression to deep vein thrombosis or thrombophlebitis. It can occur if distended varicose veins are traumatized and once this happens it is more likely to happen again. Sometimes phlebitis can progress to the deeper veins, resulting in deep vein thrombosis.

Deep Vein Thrombosis

Deep vein thrombosis is a condition, which is dangerous because it can lead to blood clots that travel to the lungs, a sometimes fatal condition. Also deep vein thrombosis in the legs can lead to a condition called postphlebitic syndrome which is characterized by chronic swelling and discomfort of the legs. For this reason it's important to treat varicose veins which can prevent this from ever happening.

Skin Problems

Varicose veins can also lead to chronic skin problems in the lower legs.

Stasis Dermatitis

Many people will develop itchiness and chronic rashes of the lower legs. This occurs because the veins do not drain the skin tissues properly allowing a buildup of toxins within the skin cells. Chronic eczema and rashes are the result.

Skin Ulceration

In the worst-case scenario leaving the veins untreated can lead to skin ulceration especially in the areas on the inside of the ankles and lower legs. In many cases these ulcers can become infected and need treatment with special dressings and antibiotics. This unfortunate condition need not occur and can be prevented if the veins are treated using one or more of the many technologies available.

Worsening Appearance

Besides the medical problems that can occur, untreated veins will undoubtedly become worse in appearance. With the increasing pressure that occurs inside the veins more spider veins and surface veins will inevitably develop.

Smaller blood vessels are usually easier to treat and can be treated with less aggressive treatments than larger blood vessels. Most of these less aggressive treatments are also less expensive so it makes sense to have veins treated when they are small and uncomplicated.

Summary

I like to tell my patients that varicose veins and spider veins should always be treated as soon as possible to avoid all of the above complications and difficulties that are associated with leaving the veins alone.

Eliminate Your Varicose and Spider Veins Now!

Dr. Peter Ursel

Chapter 7
What Are the Possible Complications of Treatment?

Most varicose vein treatments are very safe and it is unusual to see serious complications after treatment. In patients that have no medical problems it is almost unheard of to see severe complications. Most complications occur in patients that have underlying medical problems

Infection

After treatment it is possible to get an infection in the area that has been treated. Infections are more common if an excision or cut has been made such as in the surgical treatments. This is why surgery is done infrequently and less invasive treatment such as endovenous laser and injection sclerotherapy are preferred.

However it is still possible to see infections in the skin especially after injections or laser treatment. This is why it is important that your doctor always use sterile technique.

The least invasive type of treatment should always be used to minimize the risk of infection.

Signs of infection include fever, redness and swelling of the area treated. Any signs of infection should be reported to your doctor at the earliest time so treatment can be started.

Fortunately infection is extremely rare following varicose vein treatment because of today's newer less invasive procedures.

Skin Ulceration

Skin ulceration is a complication that can occur following injection sclerotherapy. It occurs if strong solutions accidentally leak out of veins that are being treated. With proper technique this complication is exceedingly rare. In addition better and safer solutions minimize the risk of this happening.

Skin ulceration and tissue damage can occur if sclerotherapy solutions are accidentally injected into arteries. This complication is exceedingly rare and occurs if caution is not taken in areas where veins and arteries are very close together.

If skin ulceration occurs it will most often heal though this can be slow. Occasionally non healing ulcers require skin grafts for full healing.

Deep Vein Thrombosis

Deep vein thrombosis is a blood clot that occurs in the deeper vein system. It is much more common following surgical stripping and ligation of veins. It occurs much less frequently following injection sclerotherapy or endo-venous procedures.

Certain patients are at much higher risk of getting deep pain thrombosis. Those at risk include people with a family history of bleeding or blood clot disorders. Patient who have a previous history of deep vein thrombosis or pulmonary embolus are at a higher risk of having another one if they have vein treatments.

There are measures that can be taken to minimize the risk of deep vein thrombosis. The first step is to avoid general anesthesia and to make sure that patients always get the least invasive treatment that will adequately treat their veins.

Early ambulation following procedures is very important to avoid deep vein thrombosis. In addition proper compression stockings will help to minimize the risk of thrombosis because they keep blood from pooling in the veins.

It's important to prevent deep vein thrombosis because it can lead to severe complications such as pulmonary embolus a condition where the blood clot moves to the lungs. This can occasionally be fatal. In addition deep vein thrombosis can lead to a condition called post phlebitic syndrome characterized by chronic swelling and valvular damage in the legs.

Allergic Reaction to Drugs

Another rare complication following varicose vein injections is allergic reactions to the solutions used. The newer solutions used nowadays are less allergenic than they used to be, however anaphylactic reactions are still possible. Properly equipped clinics can handle this complication and it's important to make sure that your clinic is so equipped.

Visual Disturbances.

Some of the newer sclerotherapy solutions can sometimes cause visual disturbances following injections. In the vast majority of cases, these symptoms are temporary and go away within a few minutes. The theory behind these visual disturbances is that the tiny bubbles that make up the solution travel to the visual part of the brain. This occurs more often in patients who have a history of migraine headache with a preceeding aura.

In addition, patients that have an abnormality in the heart where there is a small opening between chambers called patent foramen ovale (or PFO) have a higher probability of having this complication.

Blood Trapping

When veins are injected or when endovenous treatments are performed there is a possibility after the treatment that blood can get trapped in the veins. This occurs more often following sclerotherapy and is easily treated in subsequent visits to the clinic.

The treatment for this is to release the blood under local anesthetic. It's important that this is done early because it relieves discomfort and minimizes the chance of discoloration of the skin. If discoloration should occur, this is usually a temporary problem that will gradually fade over the space of 6 to 12 months.

Chemical Phlebitis

Phlebitis is inflammation of a vein. Superficial phlebitis occurs in many patients that have varicose veins before treatment. This can occur because of trauma to the legs or for no good reason at all.

Following treatment with sclerotherapy there is always inflammation in the vein but this is more of a chemical phlebitis and is completely normal. It is not dangerous and should not be mistaken for superficial phlebitis.

Skin Discoloration

Skin discoloration often occurs following vein treatments. It is more likely to occur in the summer months in patients with dark skin. It also occurs if solutions are used that are too strong or inappropriate for the type of veins being treated.

It most often goes away within 3 to 6 months though it can take longer to disappear. There are some creams that may help this complication and occasionally lasers can help. Unfortunately it is often difficult to predict which patients are going to get skin discoloration following treatment. Sun exposure can worsen pigmentation changes, so if you do have these changes it is important to stay out of the sun.

Summary

Complications are very rare following modern vein treatment. Most complications are self-limited and go away on their own following treatment. The most important thing that your doctor can do to minimize complications is to always use the least invasive and safest treatment for your particular type of vein problem

Dr. Peter Ursel

Chapter 8
How Are Leg Veins Evaluated?

Proper evaluation of leg veins is done in 3 steps. First, a thorough history of the problem is taken by the assessing doctor or nurse. A detailed history of prior vein treatments, blood clots, and medical conditions is required to determine the risk and type of future treatments.

Once this detailed history is recorded, then a proper physical examination is done, looking for the surface anatomy of veins, visible complications of the veins such as skin changes on the skin, skin ulceration and swelling of the legs. The doctor then palpates the veins to determine flow characteristics in the veins and checks the pulses to assess the health of the arterial circulation.

Once this is noted, then a special ultrasound examination is done to determine the deep vein anatomy and blood flow direction in the veins. The doctor is doing this to assess which valves are damaged and to accurately pinpoint the location of backwards blood flow.

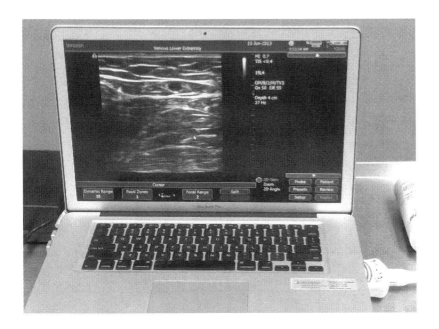

The ultrasound does 2 things. First it shows the structure of the vein system below the skin. This is very important as the abnormal veins that you see on the surface are really only the tip of the iceberg. Abnormal veins are always a sign of a problem deeper inside the body and this can only be seen with an ultrasound.

The second thing that an ultrasound shows is the direction of flow of the blood in the veins. In normal veins, the blood flows in only one direction whereas in varicose veins, the blood flows in both directions both up and down the legs. The ultrasound can detect the direction of blood flow with the color red showing blood flow in one direction and blue for the other blood flow direction.

After the physical exam and ultrasound are completed, the doctor creates a detailed map that shows both the surface and the deep vein anatomy with blood flow directions labeled. This detailed map forms the basis for all future treatments and will direct the treatment plan the doctor then creates for your particular vein problem.

What to Look For In a Vein Clinic

There are several key questions that you should have answered when you are looking for a vein clinic.

Primarily- does the clinic provide you with good educational material that you can study so you have a good understanding of the nature of your vein problem and the treatments available?

Then, is your vein problem assessed properly with a proper history, physical and ultrasound examination?

Does your doctor map out your vein problem showing both the surface and deep anatomy and present you with a treatment plan?

Are you offered a full explanation of the treatment types involved, the costs, and potential complications of treatment?

Finally, do you feel comfortable that your doctor is qualified and has proof of prior success in treating your type of vein problem?

Eliminate Your Varicose and Spider Veins Now!

Dr. Peter Ursel

Chapter 9
Other Common Questions

Question 1

Where will the blood go if a varicose vein is removed?

Dr. Ursel's Answer

This is a question that I get all the time. Most people wonder what will happen if a large vein is removed. Where will the blood go if this vein is removed? The fact is that the abnormal vein has been causing circulation problems for years and years and therefore, other channels have developed to accommodate this. When the abnormal vein is removed, the circulation always improves because the blood flow is no longer impaired or worsened by a varicose vein. Removing diseased veins always improves the circulation.

Question 2

What's it like after EVLT?

Dr. Ursel's Answer

The EVLT procedure takes about two hours and most people comment that it was a lot easier than they thought it would be. Immediately following the procedure, injections may be done in the veins below the treated vein. Following this a compression stocking is placed on the leg and you then go for a short walk.

The stocking is worn for a period of about one week and then your leg is reassessed to ensure that there are no complications and that the leg is healing well.

There is minimal discomfort in the area treated and it feels much like a pulled or strained muscle in the area that was treated. There is usually some bruising and discoloration which is usually gone within 10 days of treatment. The vein will usually appear smaller about a week after the treatment, and will steadily decrease in size as the pressure that was making it large subsides. Sometimes injections or surgery is done on the calf veins and this can speed up the results though they may cause some discoloration.

Question 3

What's it like after a vein injection treatment?

Dr. Ursel's Answer

There are different types of leg vein injections mainly divided into spider vein injections and larger vein injections.

After spider vein injections, there may be some itchiness immediately following the treatment. However there is no pain and there are really no other symptoms. A light compression stocking is frequently used after spider vein injections though this can vary depending on the severity of the problem.

After larger veins are injected with either foam or liquid sclerotherapy, the leg is initially elevated and compression is placed directly over the veins treated. This can be done with cotton or gauze pads. Following this, a stocking is placed on the leg and you will go home and likely wear the stocking for 24 to 48 hours continuously. Walking is encouraged to keep the blood flowing well in the deep vein system to prevent blood clots.

Usually a follow-up visit is arranged approximately 7 to 10 days following the initial treatment and then a series of treatments can follow after this at weekly or biweekly intervals, depending on the severity of the vein problem.

Question 4

Will pigmentation from having vein treatments go away?

Dr. Ursel's Answer

Sometimes following treatment of larger veins with injections, there is some discoloration, which can appear like brown staining over the area treated. This can happen more in individuals with darker skin, or if the area is exposed to a lot of sun after treatment.

It can also be made worse if trapped blood is left in the vein. The pigmentation occurs because the iron in the blood leaches into the skin and oxidizes (much like rust can occur on metal surfaces). The best way to prevent post treatment staining is to make sure that any trapped blood is removed and that sun exposure is avoided immediately following vein treatments.

Question 5

Is surgery still a good treatment?

Dr. Ursel's Answer

Surgery for varicose veins is less common than it used to be and is gradually being replaced by less invasive treatments. This is happening for several reasons. First, surgical treatments require more anesthesia and are thus done in hospital settings. This is not only more expensive but it also exposes patients to hospital borne infections, an unnecessary risk for someone to take for an elective procedure.

Surgery is also more risky in that infections and blood clots are more common following this type of treatment. In addition, the recovery period can be as much as six weeks after traditional stripping and ligation surgery whereas endo-venous laser procedures have a recovery period of just a week to 10 days and most people can resume work the next day.

An exception to this is the surgical procedure known as ambulatory phlebectomy, which can be done under local anesthetic and has a quick recovery. This procedure is more difficult to do and takes more time so it is gradually becoming less and less common.

Question 6

How long will it take until my legs look good again?

Dr. Ursel's Answer

The answer to this question depends both on the severity and type of veins that are being treated. With severe spider veins, sometimes 5 to 10 treatments are needed and these can be about a week apart so improvement or complete resolution of the problem could take 10 weeks or more.

With foam sclerotherapy improvement can be seen within a week, however final results could take up to 5 to 6 weeks.

With endovenous treatments, things will improve within a week and final results are usually seen at six weeks.

These are not hard and fast rules, however as a general rule with modern treatments you will see improvement within a week and complete resolution usually within a few months.

Question 7

Is vein treatment expensive?

Dr. Ursel's Answer

Modern vein treatment is not as expensive as other cosmetic treatments. Depending on the province or state you live in, treatment can range in cost from $200- $500 per treatment for sclerotherapy and $2500-$3500/leg for Endovenous procedures. Again these are just generalizations and the only way to tell for sure is to have an estimate following a proper vein evaluation.

Question 8

Is the treatment covered by insurance?

Dr. Ursel's Answer

Most vein treatments are not covered by health insurance however this varies from state-to-state and province-to-province.

Question 9

Do high heeled shoes cause leg veins?

Dr. Ursel's Answer

There is no evidence that high-heeled shoes or footwear can affect varicose veins. Wearing high heeled shoes can make it more difficult to walk and because walking is the best treatment for veins, they may have a detrimental effect.

Question 10

Can varicose veins bleed?

Dr. Ursel's Answer

Varicose veins very rarely bleed however when they do it can be quite severe. If you have veins and they start to bleed the most important thing to do is to elevate your legs and apply pressure with a towel or cloth immediately over the bleeding vein. Then, you should wrap the area with a tensor bandage.

This will stop virtually all vein bleeding until definitive treatment can be administered by a doctor or nurse.

Veins that are more likely to bleed usually are on the lower legs and will appear as very dark veins with almost transparent skin over them. These should be brought to the attention of a vein M.D. and treated preferentially before other veins are treated. If you take blood thinners and you have this type of vein problem you should have these assessed, as your risk of bleeding is even higher.

Dr. Peter Ursel

Chapter 10
Common Myths About Leg Veins

Myth 1

Vein disease is not important

Varicose vein disease does not very often cause dramatic emergencies that are life threatening. This is in sharp contrast to arterial disease which causes sudden emergencies such as heart attack and stroke which are much more dramatic and often life threatening.

However, varicose vein disease often causes chronic discomfort and problems that can greatly diminish the quality of life. Most of these problems can be tolerated for years without causing major problems. In addition, the cosmetic appearance of leg veins can have a huge negative impact on someone's self-image.

Taking these factors into consideration, it can be seen that varicose vein disease is very important; it is just less dramatic than arterial disease and therefore does not get the same attention.

Myth 2

Vein treatments cause scarring

Leg vein treatment has improved dramatically over the last 10 years. Prior to the development of endovenous procedures and injection sclerotherapy, the only treatments for varicose veins were conservative bandaging or stripping and ligation. These surgical treatments indeed caused a lot of scarring because large incisions were made and quite frequently these became infected. Now virtually all leg vein treatments are done through tiny holes made in the skin with needles so there is virtually no scarring from the procedures.

Sometimes pigmentation changes can occur after treatment, however in the worst-case scenario these are usually gone within 4 to 6 months.

The advantage of modern vein treatments is that they almost always improve leg appearance with no scarring or marks.

Myth 3

Leg pain is a normal part of aging

Many people believe that leg pain is just a normal consequence of getting older. Though it is true that arthritis and varicose veins are more common as you age, it is not true that you are necessarily going to have these problems. Regular, non-strenuous exercise, weight control and treatment of varicose veins can dramatically reduce your chances of suffering from leg pains in the future

Myth 4

Veins treatment should be done by vascular surgeons

In the past, surgery was the only option for leg vein treatment. However, in the last 20 years there has been an explosion of new minimally invasive technologies that has made it virtually unnecessary to have surgery to get rid of veins. What's important is that the doctor has training both in ultrasound investigation as well as the experience and proven success in treating a wide variety of leg vein problems. Leg vein treatment is now done by many different types of doctors, doctors from the fields of radiology, surgery, emergency and family medicines

Myth 5

Vein treatments are temporary and need to be repeated

Leg vein treatments can be extremely long-lasting and very often are permanent. This is especially true of treatments for larger blood vessels such as the greater saphenous vein and lesser saphenous vein. Generally speaking, surgical and endovenous treatments tend to be longer lasting. If injections are done on large veins there is a higher chance of recurrence.

If you suffer with spider veins, you are more likely to need treatments in the future of the same or new veins, as these veins tend to recur. Some people unfortunately have a tendency to form these veins more than others.

It is wise to keep an eye on your legs and get them assessed and re-treated if you notice any new blood vessels occurring. If you do this, you are less likely to need more expensive and invasive treatments.

Myth 6

Vein treatments can lead to more vein problems

If you have leg veins and get treatment these treatments very rarely lead to further leg vein problems. Very occasionally, injections, endovenous procedures and surgery can cause subsequent micro-vessels to form, a problem known as venous matting. This is more likely following surgery and usually subsides with time. Fortunately treatments are also available for this rare complication of treatment.

In general, leg vein treatments do not lead to more vein problems. In fact the exact opposite is true as treating one vein will most often result in the elimination of several of the branch veins coming off of it.

Myth 7

Vein treatments have a long recovery period and there is a lot of pain after

Before the modern era of vein treatment, when surgery was the only option for treatment, this was in fact true. Recovery periods of as much as six weeks were commonplace and this was often accompanied with very tight bandages and a lot of discomfort.

However nowadays, prolonged recovery is extremely rare with most people requiring stockings for just one week following the bigger procedures, and being able to return to work the day following the procedure. Things really have changed for the better!

Myth 8

Vein treatments should be done in the hospital

20 years ago before modern endovenous procedures and injection treatments were developed this may have been the case. However virtually all vein treatments are done outside of the hospital now because surgery is very rarely required.

This is now a huge advantage because general anesthetic and hospitalization can be avoided. The newer hospital acquired infections such as MRSA and C.Difficile are much less likely to occur.

Myth 9

Vein treatments are selfish and only for the vain

Some people consider cosmetic treatments for spider veins and varicose veins as being either frivolous or vain. However it must be considered that with these treatments we are only returning the appearance of the veins and legs to a normal state and are not really enhancing or changing the appearance of the legs. Furthermore leg vein treatments often dramatically improve the way that legs feel and also help to prevent complications that are often associated with varicose veins.

Spider vein treatments can also make the legs feel a lot better as well improving the appearance of the legs. Finally when compared to the cost of other cosmetic treatments leg vein treatments are quite affordable.

Myth 10

Vein treatments are painful

Modern treatment technology has dramatically decreased the amount of pain that is experienced with leg vein treatment. For example when doing endovenous laser treatment there is only the slight discomfort from injecting a small amount of weak local anesthetic. The laser is not uncomfortable as the local anesthetic used completely numbs the leg.

Leg vein injections are virtually painless and made even more comfortable with the use of topical numbing creams or cooling devices. There is no pain after injection treatments, except maybe a small amount of tenderness over the vein injection sites.

Older treatments such as stripping and ligation can be quite uncomfortable (especially following the procedure) however these treatments are very rarely used now so this is no longer much of an issue.

In general most leg vein treatments are virtually painless and the technological developments that are occurring are improving this all the time.

Eliminate Your Varicose and Spider Veins Now!

Chapter 11
Case Studies Of Successful Treatments

Case Study 1
Varicose Veins On Back Of Thigh

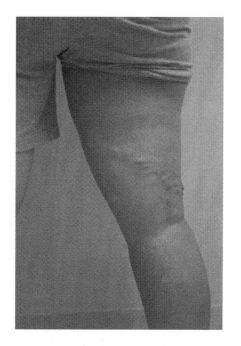
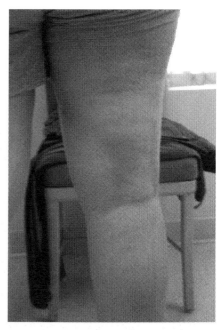

Before **After**

The Story

This 35 year old ladies leg veins really became quite painful and evident after having her third child. She was otherwise very healthy and had no previous history of vein treatments or surgery.

Evaluation

When she came in for her assessment the physical exam showed that she had no skin complications from her veins and that she had no other leg symptoms.

Her ultrasound exam revealed poorly functioning valves at the top of her greater saphenous vein with backwards flow to the surface veins on her posterior thigh.

The Treatment

After discussing the options with her, we decided to go ahead with endovenous laser treatment (EVLT) and also to remove the lower part of the vein with ambulatory phlebectomy.

This was all done in one 2 hour session with resulting good cosmetic results and complete resolution of her leg swelling and pain. She wore a stocking for one week and was able to return to her usual activities almost immediately.

Eliminate Your Varicose and Spider Veins Now!

Case Study 2
Reticular Veins

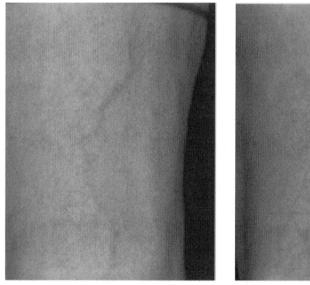 

Before   **After**

The Story

This 44-year-old lady did not like the appearance of the veins on the back of her knee. There is no pain with these veins and she had no previous treatment. She was otherwise well.

Evaluation

Her physical examination showed these green or reticular veins in the area on the back of her knee as well as some accompanying spider veins. Her ultrasound examination was entirely normal.

The Treatment

Initially the reticular veins or green veins were treated with foam sclerotherapy. After three weeks the veins were reevaluated and the reticular veins as well as most of the spider veins had disappeared. The spider veins were then injected with a weaker solution and then completely resolved.

Re-evaluation was arranged in approximately one year for follow up and ensure that the good results are maintained.

Case Study 3

Popliteal Veins

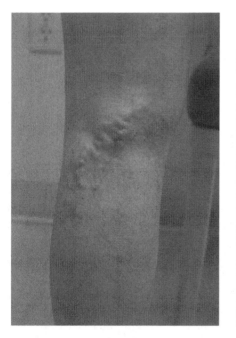 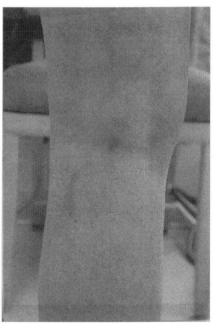

Before   **After**

The Story

This 37 year old lady has suffered from varicose veins and spider veins on the back of her knee or the popliteal area. She has had no other treatments for the veins however she now is getting tired of their appearance and the aching. As well, she is worried that they are going to bleed if they get bumped.

Evaluation

These veins are protruding and unsightly but are not really a danger. There are no signs of vein complications such as skin changes or ulceration. Her ultrasound exam show poorly functioning valves in her posterior thigh veins, however the vein is very bent and tortuous.

The Treatment

The ideal treatment for this size of vein would be endovenous laser combined with sclerotherapy of the smaller spider veins. However, because the deep feeding vein is very bent, it would not be possible to put the laser inside the vein so it was elected to do sclerotherapy on this patient. She required 5 visits with very good results. The photo shows some discoloration at 4 months, however this was completely gone one year after treatment. She will require follow up yearly to treat any minor new veins, however she is now free of the large veins.

Case Study 4

Spider Veins

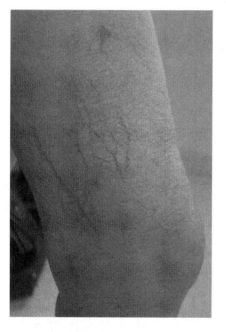

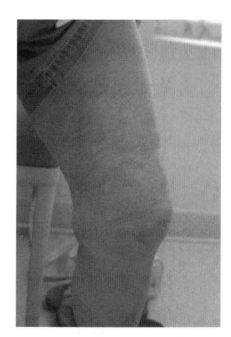

Before **After**

The Story

This 72 year old lady has had spider veins for over 30 years and finally decided that she wanted to be rid of them. She had no other treatments for them other than covering them up with makeup. She is otherwise healthy and has no other symptoms from her leg veins

Evaluation

Her physical exam reveals no obvious varicose veins however, she does have some spider veins that are not bulging at all.

Her ultrasound examination is completely normal and there are no obvious abnormal valves seen.

The Treatment

This lady had a series of spider vein injections coupled with injections of liquid sclerosant into the feeding reticular veins (these are only visible with a special vein light) Each treatment was approximately one week apart and five treatments were required. There were no pigmentation changes from the treatments and she feels her veins are about 80% improved. She will return in about one year for reassessment and probably one treatment.

Case Study 5
Tiny Spider Veins On Ankle

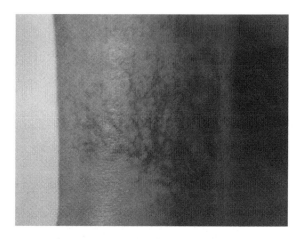

Before

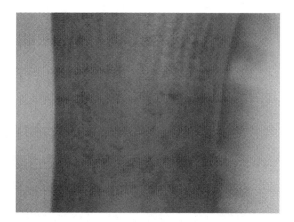

After

The Story

This 35-year-old lady has no history of varicose veins however she noticed that she has this large area of spider veins that are very tightly knit on her ankle. These have been there for years however they have recently become a lot worse. She has no history of previous treatments and is otherwise healthy.

Evaluation

Her physical examination showed that she had no other areas on her legs with visible veins. Her skin shows no other changes related to varicose vein disease. Her ultrasound examination was entirely normal.

The Treatment

Initially she was treated with injection sclerotherapy. These treatments were ineffective so it was elected to try treatment with broadband light therapy or BBL. After one treatment, she had dramatic improvement of these veins and it was decided that this was enough. Two years later no recurrence of these veins occured and she was instructed to return for treatment if there is any recurrence.

Eliminate Your Varicose and Spider Veins Now!

Chapter 12
Summary

Varicose veins and spider veins are now very treatable for just about everyone that suffers with them. Modern medical technology has made it possible to have treatments that work quickly with minimal side effects and almost no down time

To get great results, it is important to first have a proper evaluation, which includes both a physical and ultrasound exam. Once these have been done your vein map is created, and then a step-by-step plan is put together to treat the underlying cause of your vein problem. Multiple treatment modalities are frequently used and sometimes several visits are required to achieve optimal results.

Remember, that you now have little to fear with modern vein treatments. Surgical horror stories are mostly a thing of the past. Hooray for modern vein technology and treatments!

About Dr. Ursel

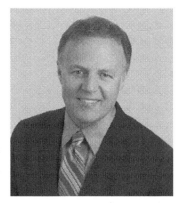

Dr Peter Ursel has been treating leg vein patients in Lindsay Ontario for almost 20 years. He was initially a family and emergency physician and early in his career discovered that there was a need in his area for outpatient vein treatments.

At the time, there was no formal training available. After extensive research and over many years, Doctor Ursel assembled the finest treatments available and brought them to Lindsay.

In 2002 there was no effective outpatient treatment available for large varicose veins, so Dr. Ursel went to New York City and learned how to do the EVLT or Endovenous Laser Treatment from Dr. Robert Min, one of the treatments developers. Since that time, he has helped thousands of people eliminate their unsightly leg veins.

Dr. Ursel can be reached at his clinic in Lindsay at 705-328-1747 or Online at www.doctorursel.com

Eliminate Your Varicose and Spider Veins Now!

Dr. Peter Ursel

Reports From
Dr. Ursel's Patients

Having a large vein procedure, I appreciated walking out of the office, not being in a hospital, awake through the procedure, recovery fast and painless. Didn't lose any time from my job. They always explained what they were doing.
It was an excellent procedure – I can't say enough. The clinic was very clean and sterile. Dr. Ursel and staff were wonderful! It was a great feeling to see the difference from before and after. Dr. Ursel and staff know what they are doing.
M.V.

After a consultation with a Toronto vascular surgeon, I was advised that surgical ligation and stripping was too risky at my age. Fortunately, I learned that EVLT procedure by Dr. Ursel could safely remove varicose veins. All of the required procedures were carried out by Dr. Ursel and his support staff in a courteous and professional manner. I can highly recommend Dr. Ursel for the treatment of varicose vein problems that are not available by conventional methods.
B.C.

The vein procedure was quick, painless and friendly. I have recommended your service to several of my friends and acquaintances who have similar leg problems.
E.L.

The staff was friendly and made me feel at ease. The doctor and nurse were very professional but at the same time, very caring and considerate. I recommend laser treatments, if possible, it is not a painful procedure and you can continue your normal activities – within reason.
E.S.

I had pain in my lower leg. It was worth paying to get this procedure done. Thanks for my new leg!
G.L.

The doctor makes you feel relaxed, explains everything well, receptionist very nice too. Appreciate the sclerotherapy on legs. Will give me more confidence when wearing shorts, skirts, bathing suit.
A.K.

Eliminate Your Varicose and Spider Veins Now!

Made in the USA
Lexington, KY
13 September 2019